Firefly
Night

Written by Evanne Beth Jordan

Illustrated by Mary Ruth Patchin

Interdimensional Press
Brentwood, CA 94513

First Published by Interdimensional Press, December 2010

ISBN: 978-0-9827753-4-9

Library of Congress Control Number: 201094317

Printed in the United States of America,
La Vergne, Tennessee

This book is printed on acid-free paper.

Firefly Night

Dedicated to
Michael for his love and support

Thank you to
Gina Lorenzo - Editor Extraordinaire

Mary Ruth Patchin - Illustrator Beyond Compare

Patricia and Byron McCulley -
Interdimensional Press
For making my dreams come true

The Lafayette Child Day School
For their enthusiasm and support

My friends and family

And to B.J. and Sydney

May you all have many more Firefly Nights!
-Evanne

To Mom, Dad, and Katie
Thank you for your never-ending support!
-Mary

One warm summer eve,

beneath a night sky,

Ajay and Sidney decided to try

and catch more than one

of the bright fireflies.

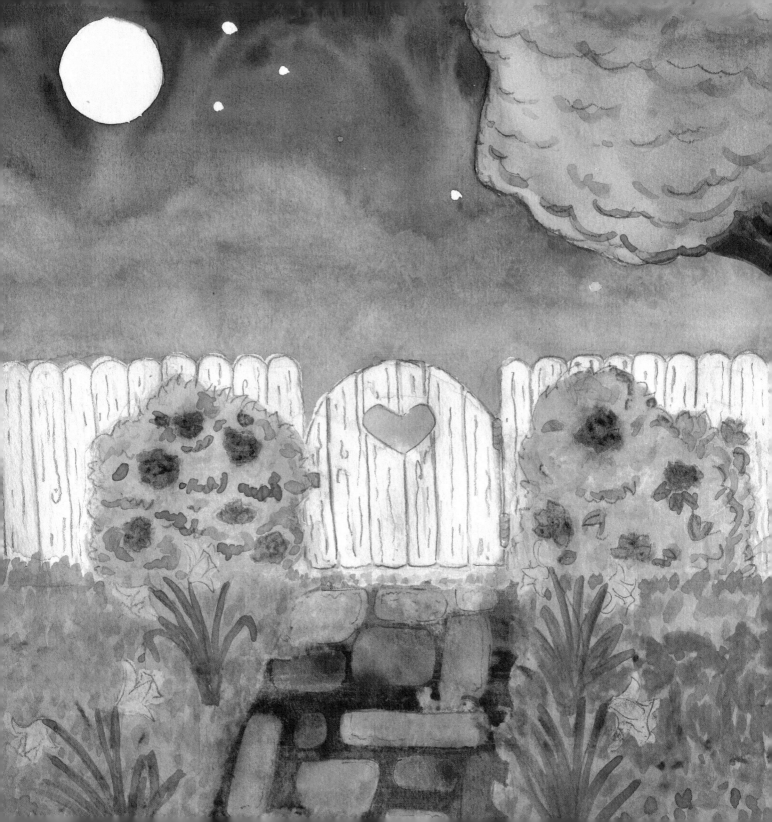

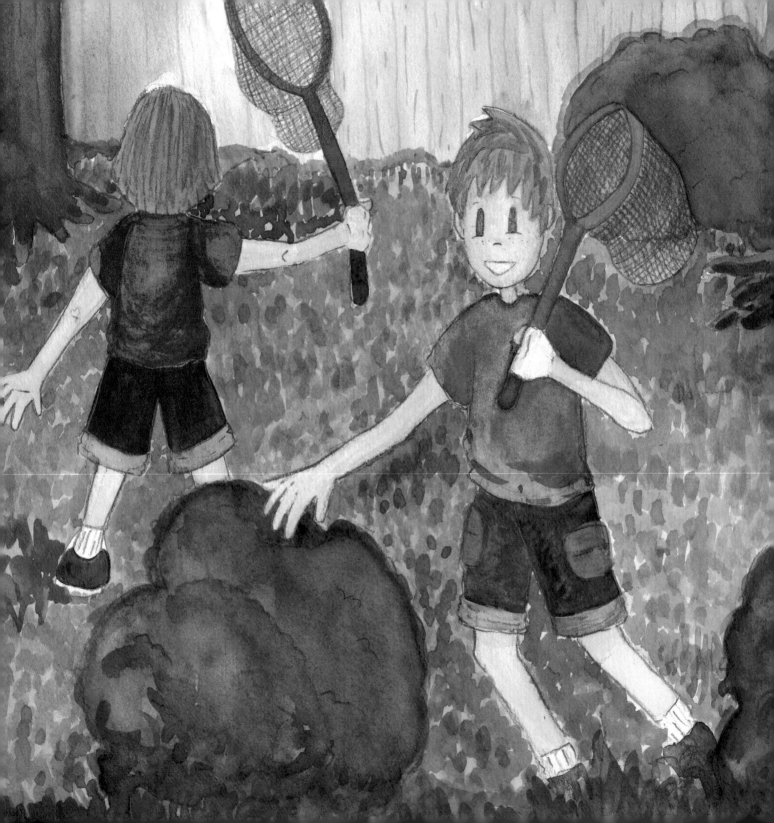

They brought out their nets, jar and bug-catching potions and started by making some bug-catching motions.

One tired firefly,
flying all alone,
was the first to be put into
their own bug home.

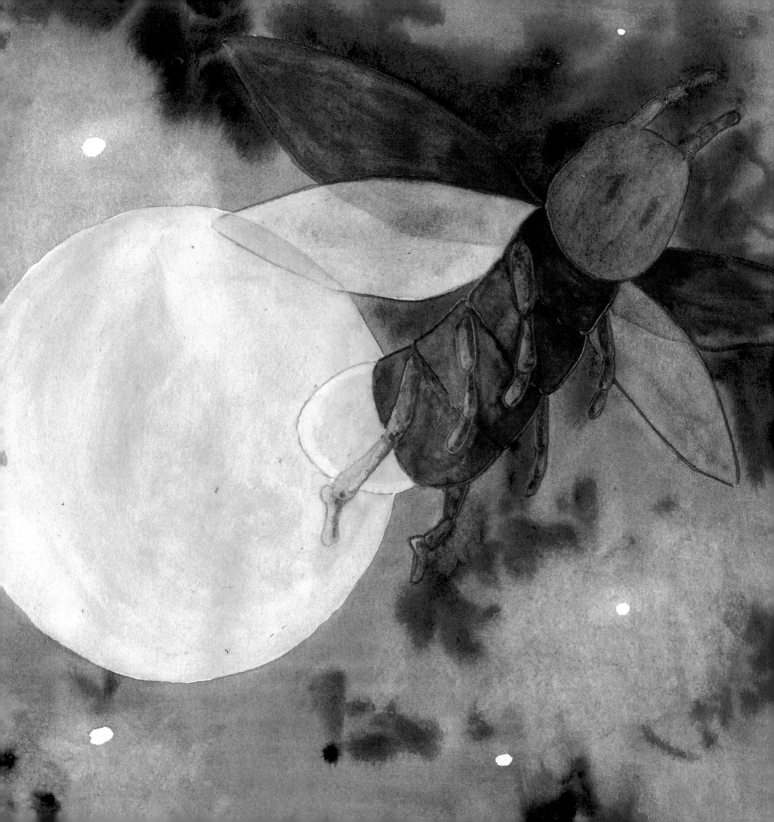

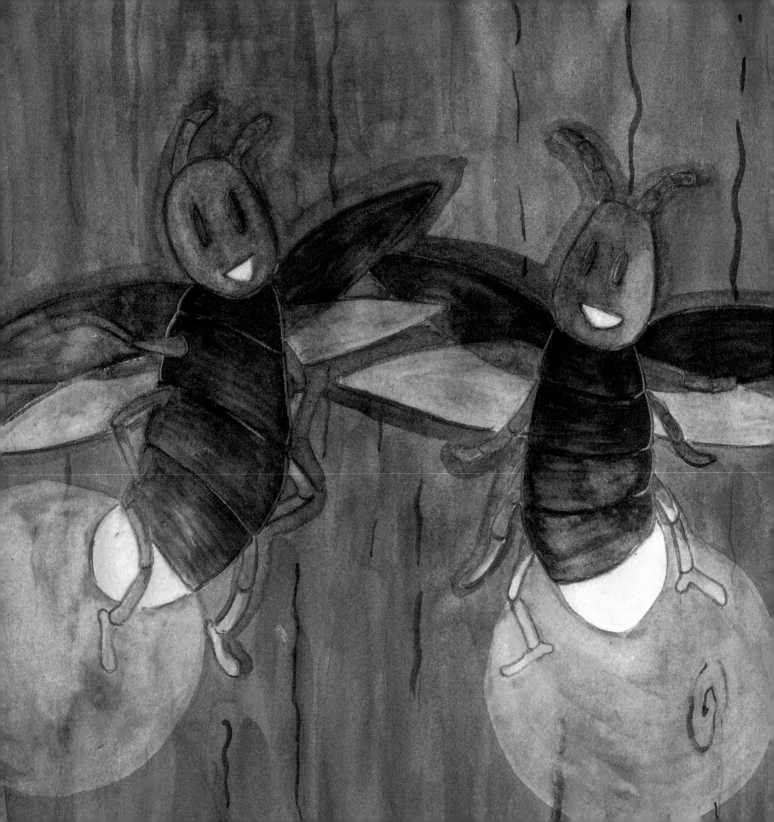

Two friendly fireflies,

chatting near a tree,

were the next to be sitting

in the jar on momma's knee.

Three lady fireflies,

all dressed to go out,

ended up in Sidney's net

and began to hum and pout.

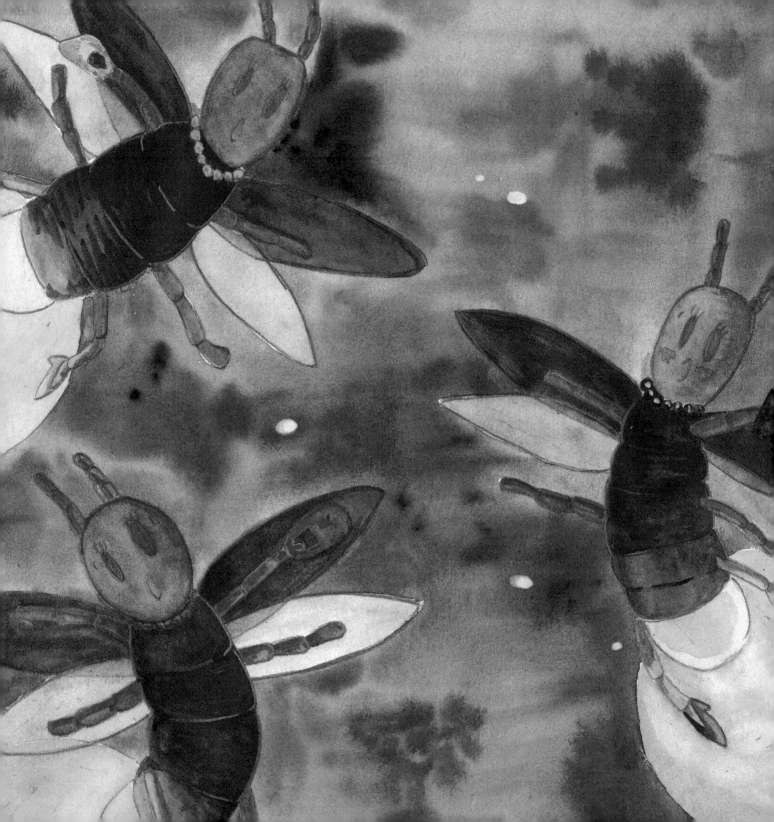

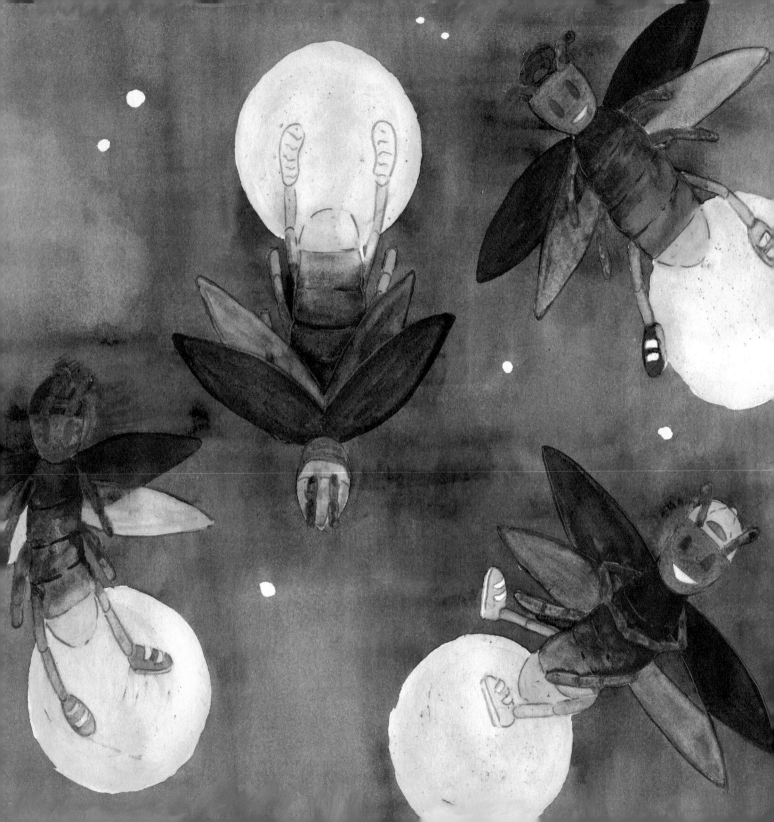

Four boy fireflies,

Iz, Biz, Ike and Willy,

were caught as they dived

in the air and got silly.

Five baby fireflies,

crying for their mommas,

flew into the jar

while wearing their pajamas.

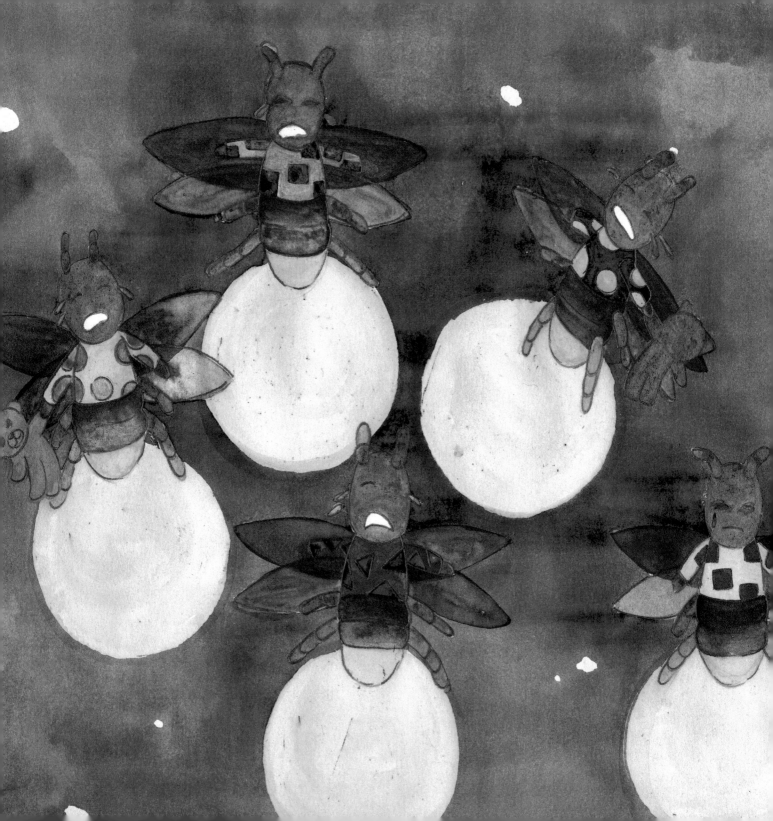

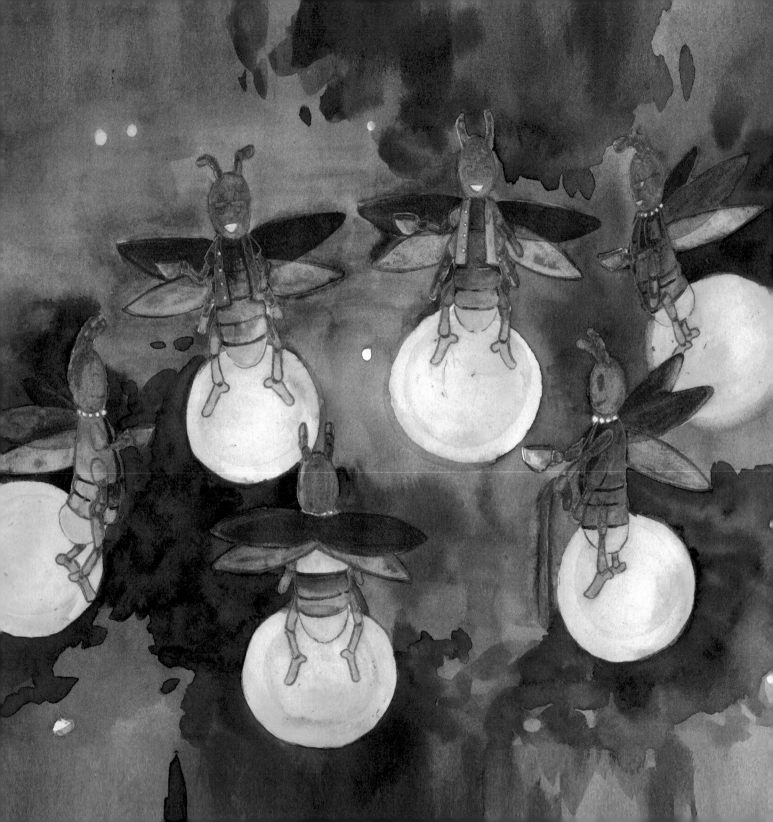

Six grandma fireflies,

sipping mint leaf tea,

were captured by Ajay who

shouted with glee,

"I am King of the Fireflies!"

"Look at me! Look at me!"

Seven smart fireflies

hid under the car,

but Sidney swooped in

and put them in the jar.

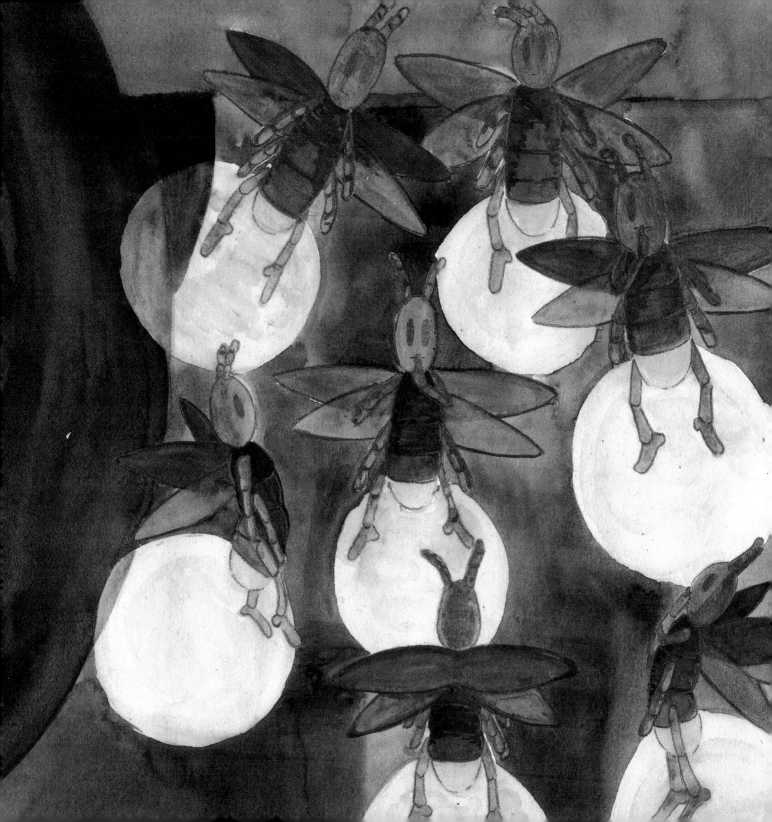

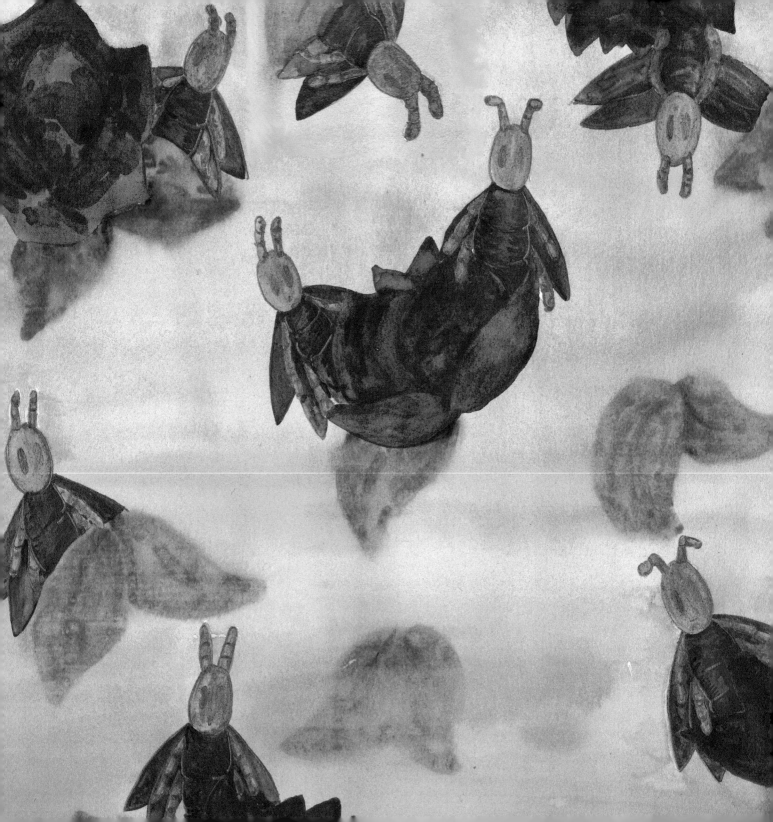

By this time it was dark
and getting quite late,
but it did not stop Ajay
who found the next eight
in the lovely rosebushes,
behind the front gate.

Not to be outdone,

Sidney went looking

and after some time,

caught nine more cooking

some firefly stew,

and she said with a grin,

"I can catch some more!"

"I think I will win!"

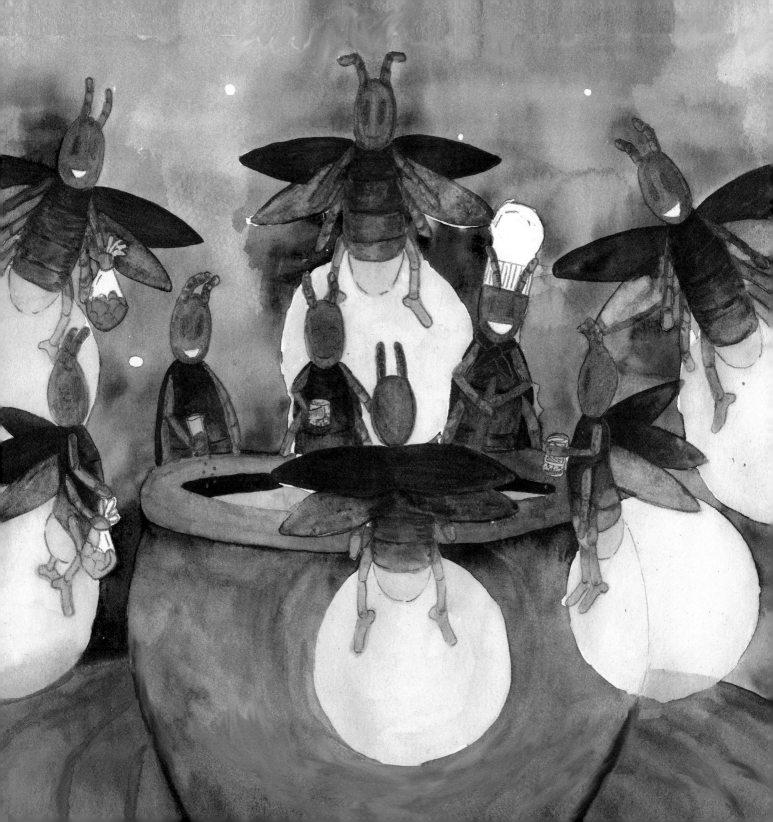

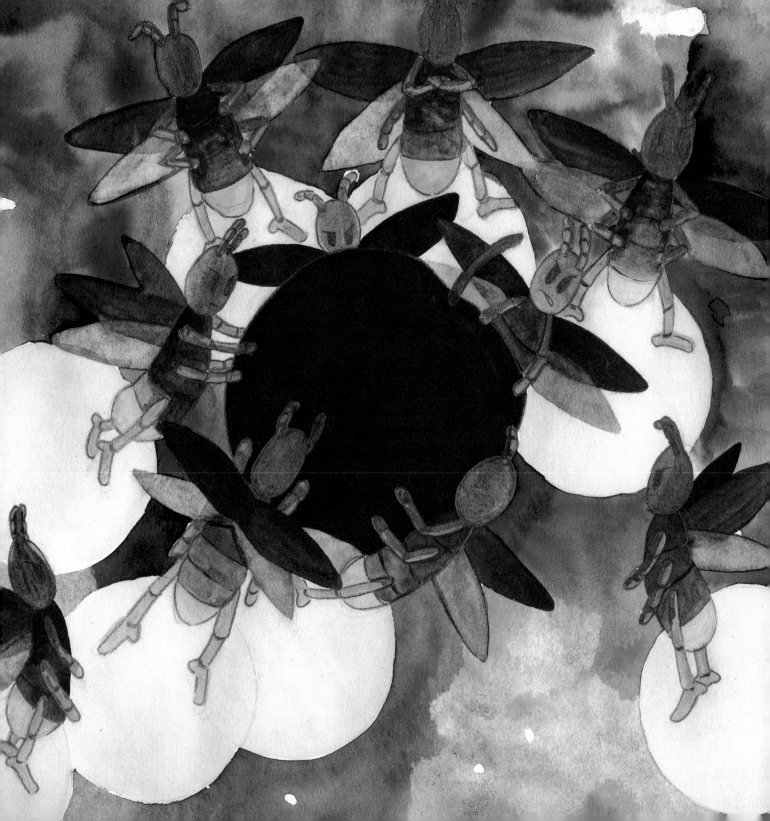

Just then from a distance

there came quite a hum

as ten tired fireflies

fought over a plum.

Ajay and Sidney

decided to hurry

to capture these ten

before they could scurry.

Now all at once,

the jar was aglow

as all of the fireflies

made a light show.

The light was so clear,

so great and so bright,

that the one little jar

lit up the whole night.

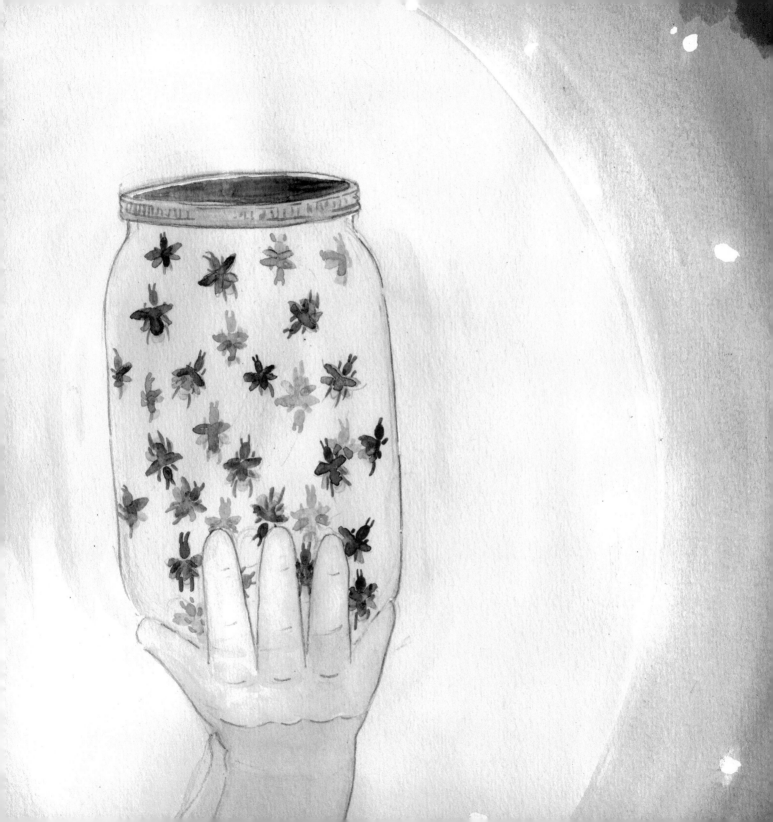

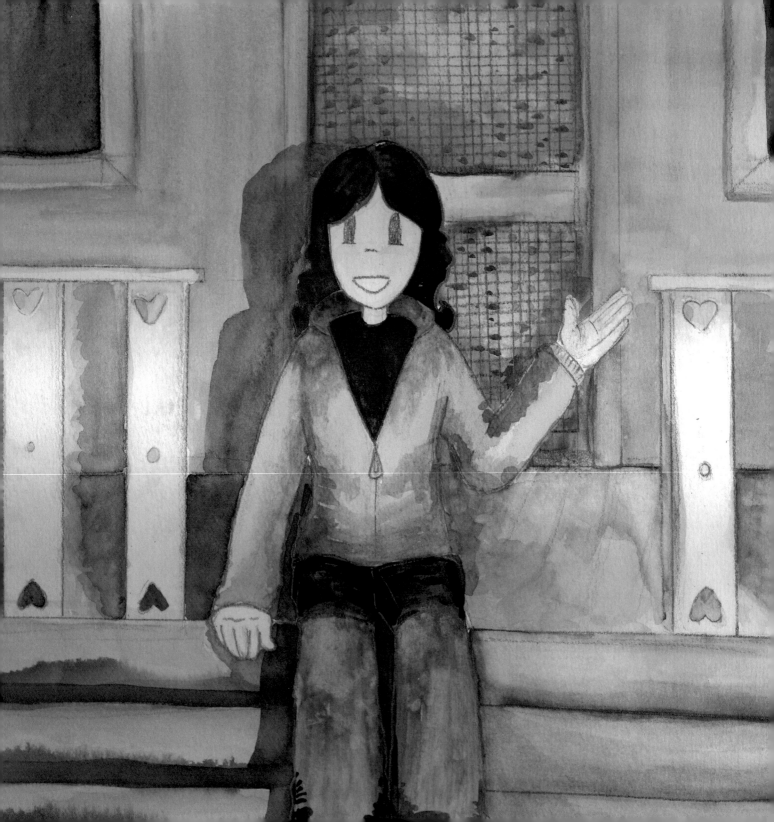

But Momma looked worried and asked, "Do you think it is right to keep all those fireflies locked up for the night?"

Ajay and Sydney

decided that night

to do the one thing

that they knew was just right.

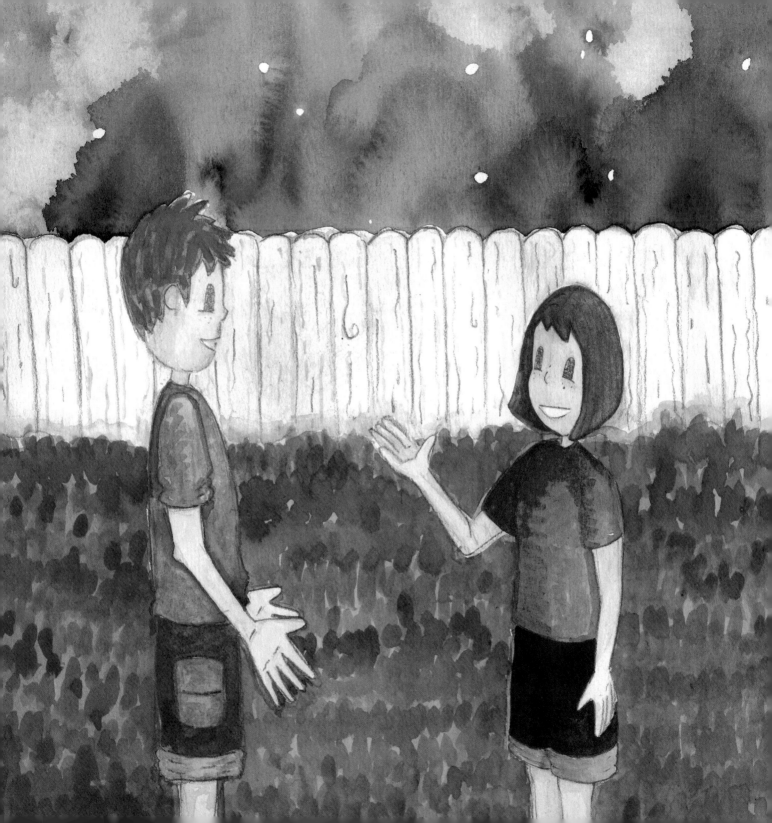

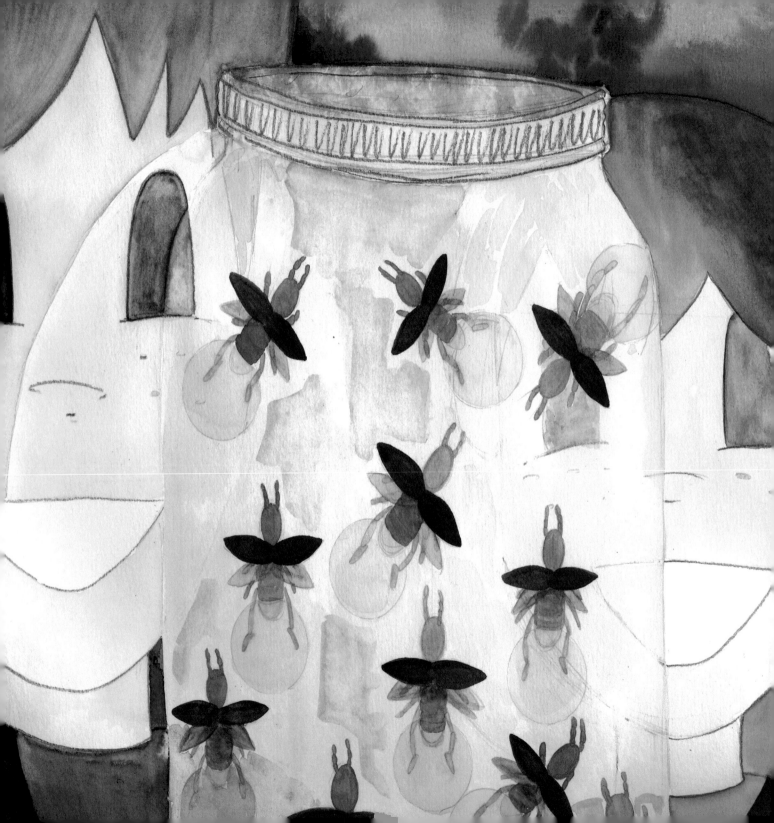

Then the children that moment
did solemnly agree
"We are King and Queen
of Fireflies, and will
create harmony."

"We have captured so many,
and will now let them free!"
Then the fireflies flew away
one two three!

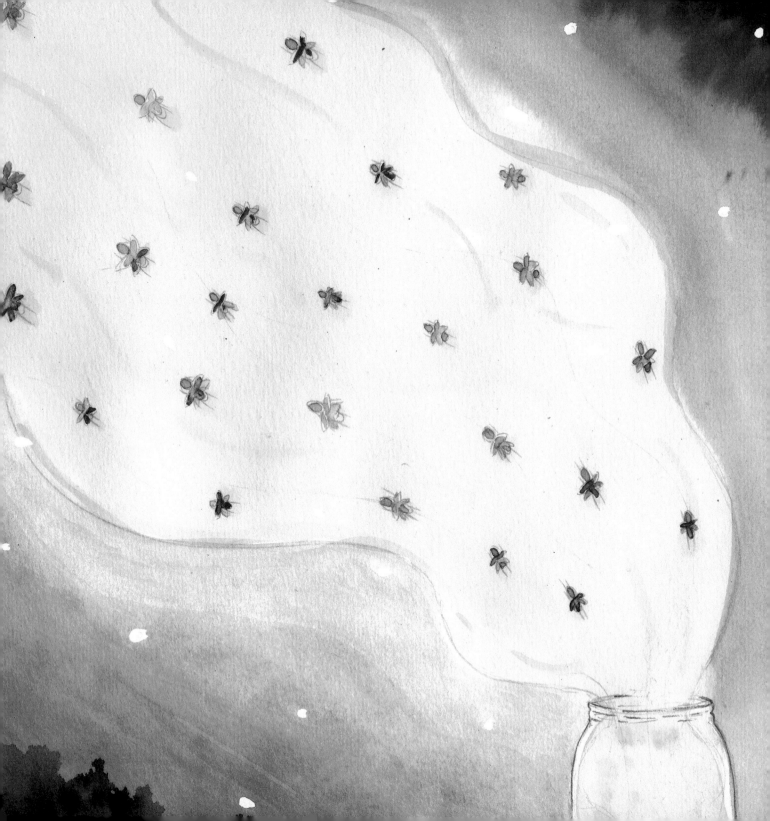

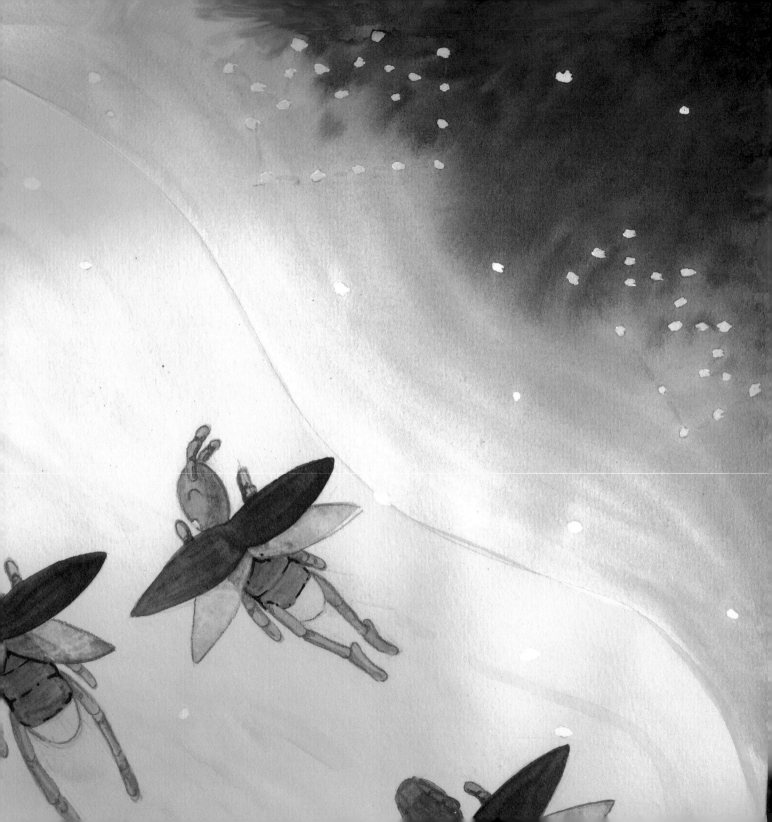

Their yellow lights were blinking,

and flashing with gold.

One could see in their trails

the message they told.

"We met the Royal Family

and as you can see

they were noble and kind

and they set us all free!"

Our tale has been told,

fireflies now are free,

but if you are not sleepy

count fireflies again with me!

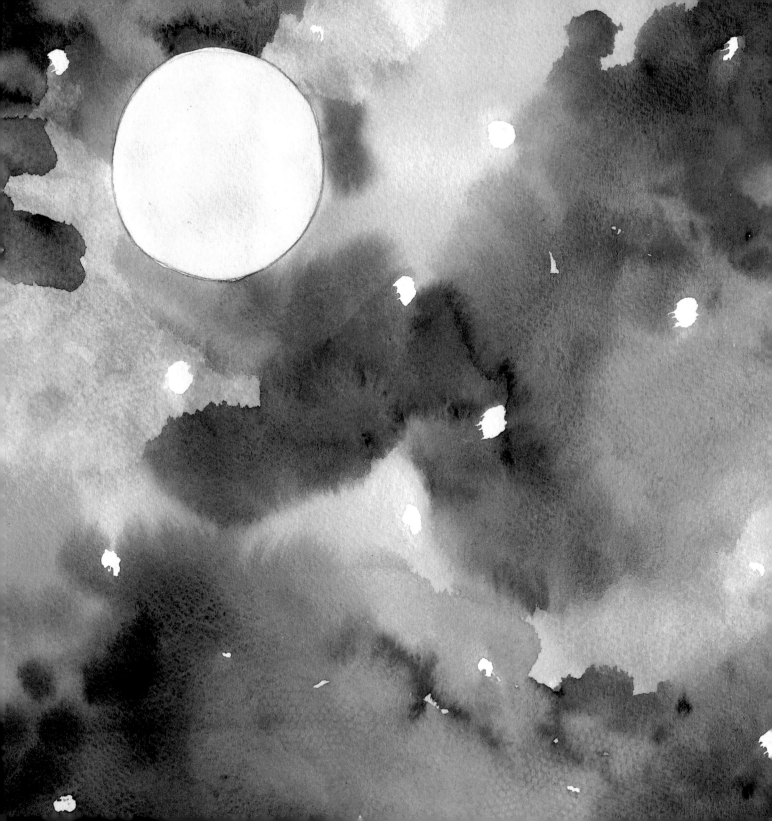

$9.99

7-12

T 567622

CPSIA information can be obtained
at www.ICGtesting.com
Printed in the USA
LVIC080821130612

285903LV00003B